The Constipation Solution

A Comprehensive Guide to Digestive Health

Abhiroop Bhattacharyya

Constipation can be an uncomfortable and frustrating condition affecting millions worldwide. Left untreated, it can cause various physical and mental health issues, including bloating, abdominal pain, hemorrhoids, anxiety, and depression.

If you're struggling with constipation, you're not alone. The good news is that you can make numerous natural remedies, medical treatments, and lifestyle changes to manage and even prevent constipation.

This book is designed to provide a comprehensive guide to relieving constipation. You'll learn about the causes and symptoms of constipation and the most effective natural and medical treatments available. We'll also discuss lifestyle changes you can make to promote regular bowel movements and prevent constipation from recurring.

Whether you're experiencing occasional constipation or chronic symptoms, this book will give you the knowledge and tools to control your digestive health. So, let's begin the journey to better bowel movements and a happier, healthier you.

Table of Content

Understanding Constipation

Constipation afflicts individuals regardless of their gender or age. It entails rare bowel movements, arduous stool passage, and a sense of incomplete defecation. Occasional constipation is usual and, more often than not, isn't cause for concern. Prolonged constipation, on the other hand, induces discomfort, agony, and other (sometimes deadly) health complications. Comprehending the causes, symptoms, and treatment alternatives is vital for optimal digestive health.

The digestive system is a labyrinthine amalgamation of organs and tissues that synergize to break down food particles and absorb nutrients. Disruptions to this intricate system could cause various digestive predicaments, including constipation. Although sedentary lifestyles and dietary choices could contribute to constipation, medical conditions like hypothyroidism, IBS, and Parkinson's disease could also cause constipation.

This article will review the definition of constipation and its effects on the body. It will also delve into the usual causes of constipation, encompassing lifestyle choices and medical conditions. Furthermore, we will probe the symptoms of constipation in men, women, and children. Lastly, we will discuss the diverse treatment alternatives for constipation, depending on the underlying cause.

Remember, by acquiring a profound comprehension of constipation and its causes; individuals could adopt proactive measures to prevent and manage this common digestive issue, improving their overall well-being and digestive health.

What is constipation, and How Does it Affect the Body?

Constipation is a daunting digestive dilemma marked by the colon's unquenchable thirst for water from consumed sustenance. When bowel movements become infrequent or arduous, one is deemed constipated. This results in the formation of obstinate, parched, and arduous-to-pass feces.

Whether acute or chronic, constipation is determined by the duration of its persistence. Acute constipation, a sudden onset, typically lasts a brief period. Chronic constipation, on the other hand, is when one experiences fewer than three bowel movements per week for several weeks or more.

Common Causes of Constipation

The causes of constipation, attributed to lifestyle factors and medical conditions, are myriad. Here are some of the most common:

1. Lifestyle Factors

It's critical to note that lifestyle factors can interact with one another and contribute to constipation. For instance, a diet low in fiber and high in processed foods combined with a sedentary lifestyle can augment the risk of constipation. Similarly, stress can lead to changes in diet and hydration, further exacerbating the issue.

2. Inadequate fiber intake

Fiber plays a pivotal role in sustaining regular bowel movements. A diet low in fiber can lead to constipation. Fiber-rich foods encompass fruits, vegetables, whole grains, legumes, nuts, and seeds.

3. Sedentary lifestyle

Lack of physical activity can decelerate the digestive system, leading to constipation. Regular exercise, such as walking or jogging, can help stimulate the digestive system and promote regular bowel movements.

4. Ignoring the urge to defecate

Disregarding the urge to defecate can lead to constipation, as stools can become harder and more arduous to pass over time.

5. Not drinking enough water

Hydration is key to keeping stools soft and easy to pass. A lack of water can lead to dehydration and constipation.

6. Traveling

Alterations in routine, diet, and hydration during travel can disrupt bowel movements and lead to constipation.

7. Stress

Chronic stress can precipitate constipation, as it can impact the functioning of the digestive system.

8. Medications

Certain medications, such as opioids, antidepressants, and antacids, can cause constipation as a side effect.

To prevent constipation caused by lifestyle factors, making changes that ameliorate overall health and well-being is crucial. Such changes may include:

Incorporating more fruits, vegetables, whole grains, legumes, nuts, and seeds into the diet can help prevent constipation.

10.   Drinking enough water

Staying hydrated can help keep stools soft and easy to pass.

11.   Exercising regularly

Regular exercise can help stimulate the digestive system and promote regular bowel movements.

12.   Going to the bathroom when needed

Responding promptly to the urge to defecate can help prevent constipation.

13.   Managing stress

Finding ways to manage stress, such as meditation, yoga, or counseling, can help prevent constipation.

14.   Being mindful of medications

Being cognizant of medications that can cause constipation as a side effect and consulting a healthcare provider for alternative options can help prevent constipation.

By implementing these lifestyle changes, individuals can help prevent constipation and promote overall digestive health. However, it is vital to note that medical attention should be sought if constipation persists despite lifestyle changes or is accompanied by other symptoms.

Medical Conditions

Medical maladies wield a hefty influence in evoking constipation. Recognizing the medical afflictions that can prompt constipation is pivotal for accurate diagnosis and treatment. Rectifying the underlying ailment can ameliorate constipation.

This section will delve into some of the prevalent medical conditions that can contribute to constipation and the treatments available to assuage this gastrointestinal issue.

1.   Irritable bowel syndrome (IBS)

IBS is a prevalent digestive disorder that affects the large intestine. It is a chronic condition that can elicit a medley of symptoms, including constipation. IBS-related constipation may be accompanied by abdominal pain, bloating, and gas.

The exact cause of IBS is abstruse, but it may be associated with anomalous contractions of the muscles in the intestine or hypersensitivity to certain foods or stress.

2.   Diabetes

Diabetes is a chronic condition that affects the way the body processes blood sugar. Over time, diabetes can inflict damage to the nerves that govern the digestive system, leading to constipation. Additionally, some diabetes medications can induce constipation as a side effect.

3.   Hypothyroidism

Hypothyroidism is a condition where the thyroid gland does not secrete enough thyroid hormone. This can result in slowing down the digestive system and cause constipation. Furthermore, hypothyroidism can cause fatigue, weight gain, and hypersensitivity to cold.

4.   Multiple sclerosis (MS)

MS is a condition that impacts the nervous system, including the nerves that govern the digestive system. MS-related constipation may be due to nerve damage that affects the functioning of the digestive system. Other symptoms of MS may include muscle weakness, fatigue, and difficulty walking.

5.   Parkinson's disease

Parkinson's disease is a condition that affects movement and can also impact the digestive system, leading to constipation.

Parkinson's disease-related constipation may be due to muscle stiffness and decreased mobility. Other symptoms of Parkinson's disease may include tremors, rigidity, and difficulty with balance and coordination.

6.   Colorectal cancer

Colorectal cancer is a type of cancer that affects the colon or rectum. One of the symptoms of colorectal cancer can be constipation and other symptoms such as abdominal pain, bleeding, and weight loss.

Colorectal cancer is often treatable if detected early, so it is imperative to seek medical attention if you are experiencing persistent constipation or other symptoms.

7.   Inflammatory bowel disease (IBD)

IBD is a group of conditions that cause inflammation in the digestive system, including Crohn's disease and ulcerative colitis. IBD-related constipation may be due to inflammation in the colon or rectum, leading to difficulty passing stool. Other symptoms of IBD may include abdominal pain, diarrhea, and weight loss.

8.   Diverticulitis

Diverticulitis is a condition where small pockets in the colon become infected or inflamed. This can lead to constipation and other symptoms such as abdominal pain and fever. Diverticulitis is more prevalent in older adults and can often be treated with antibiotics and dietary changes.

9.   Pregnancy

Pregnancy can lead to constipation due to hormonal changes that decelerate the digestive system and pressure on the intestines from the growing uterus. Constipation is a common complaint during pregnancy and can often be managed with dietary changes and increased physical activity.

10.   Aging

The digestive system may slow down as individuals age, leading to constipation. In addition, medications commonly used by older adults can cause constipation as a side effect.

Older adults may also be more susceptible to medical conditions that can cause constipation, such as Parkinson's disease and hypothyroidism.

It is crucial to note that constipation can also be a symptom of more serious medical conditions, such as intestinal obstruction, bowel cancer, or nerve damage. Medical attention should be sought immediately if constipation is persistent or accompanied by other symptoms, such as severe abdominal pain or bleeding.

Signs and Symptoms of Constipation

Constipation affects people of all ages and genders, but some groups may be more susceptible than others. Here are some signs and symptoms associated with constipation in men, women, and children:

Men

- **Exerting themselves during bowel movements**: Men may find themselves straining to push out stool, a telltale sign of constipation.

- **Feeling incomplete after evacuation:** After evacuating, men with constipation may feel as though they have not entirely emptied their bowels.

- **Abdominal discomfort or agony**: Constipation can cause abdominal agony or discomfort, making men feel bloated and uneasy.

- **Reduced appetite:** Men may feel less hungry due to constipation, which can make them feel full and uncomfortable.

- **Nausea or vomiting:** In severe cases, constipation can cause men to feel nauseous or even vomit.

Women

- **Pelvic distress or torment:** Constipation can cause women to experience pelvic distress or torment.

- **Painful intercourse:** Women with constipation may experience painful intercourse, making it difficult to enjoy intimacy.

- **Rectal bleeding or hemorrhoids:** Straining during bowel movements can cause women to suffer from rectal bleeding or hemorrhoids.

- **Fatigue:** Women may feel fatigued and unwell due to constipation, which can cause them to feel uncomfortable.

- **Hormonal shifts during menstruation or pregnancy:** Hormonal shifts during menstruation or pregnancy can slow down the digestive system, leading to constipation in women.

Children

- **Rare bowel movements:** Children may experience infrequent bowel movements and have trouble passing hard stool when constipated.

- **Abdominal pain or discomfort:** Constipation can cause children to feel abdominal pain or discomfort.

- **Refusal to eat or drink:** Children may refuse to eat or drink due to the discomfort caused by constipation.

- **Stool withholding behavior:** Some children may deliberately withhold stool, leading to constipation.

- **Stool incontinence:** In severe cases, constipation can cause stool incontinence, where children may involuntarily defecate due to a buildup of stool in the colon.

The National Institute of Diabetes and Digestive and Kidney Diseases (NIDDK) estimates that 16% of American adults suffer from constipation, with women and older adults being more susceptible to the condition.

Children can also experience constipation, with up to 30% of them suffering from it at some point in their lives.

Natural remedies for constipation

Constipation plagues people of all ages, an affliction causing infrequent bowel movements, arduous stool passage, and bowel strain. Though occasional constipation may be commonplace, the chronic variety births discomfort, bloating, and further complications.

Luckily, a plethora of natural remedies exist to alleviate constipation and promote regular bowel movements. From altering your diet to exercise, herbal remedies, supplements, and stress management techniques, these remedies can work wonders when incorporated into your daily routine.

This blog post will delve into each remedy in intricate detail, offering tips on how to utilize them best. Whether you're hit by occasional or chronic constipation, you can find relief via these remedies and improve your digestive health.

With no further ado, let's explore the natural remedies that foster regular bowel movements and alleviate constipation.

Dietary Changes to Promote Regular Bowel Movements

Dietary changes are one of the most effective, easiest, and natural ways to alleviate constipation. You can promote regular bowel movements and improve your digestive health by incorporating certain foods and eliminating others. Here are some tips:

1.   Increase fiber intake

Fiber is an essential nutrient for digestive health and has been proven to add bulk to the stool, making it easier to pass. It also helps promote steady bowel movements by stimulating the muscles in the large intestines.

Some excellent fiber sources include legumes, vegetables, whole grains, and fruits. Below is a brief list of some high-fiber foods you should consider adding to your diet:

- Whole-grain bread and cereals

- Brown rice

- Quinoa

- Lentils and beans

- Fresh fruits and vegetables

Experts recommend gradually increasing your fiber intake to avoid bloating and discomfort. Aim to boost your daily fiber intake by 5 grams per day until you hit the recommended intake of 25-30 grams per day.

2.   Stay hydrated

Drinking enough water is also quite essential for digestive health as it helps keep the stool soft, making it easy to pass. When one is dehydrated, the body absorbs more water from the colon, making it harder and more difficult to pass stool.

As a general rule, aim to drink at least eight glasses of water per day to help prevent constipation.

Processed foods are often low in fiber and high in salt, sugar, and unhealthy fats, which can, in turn, contribute to constipation and other digestive issues. As an alternative, consider focusing on whole foods like fruits, vegetables, whole grains, and lean protein (as indicated above.)

4.   Eat prunes or drink prune juice

Prunes are naturally existing laxatives that have been proven to help relieve constipation. They are high in fiber and contain sorbitol, which is a sugar alcohol that can help soften stool and promote bowel movements.

Experts recommend adding a few prunes to your diet or drinking a glass of prune juice each day to help prevent or alleviate constipation.

5.   Avoid dairy products

Some individuals are sensitive to lactose, the kind of sugar found in dairy products. If these individuals consume the sugar, it can cause constipation. If you suspect dairy products could contribute to your constipation, consider eliminating them from your diet for several weeks to see if your symptoms improve.

These dietary changes should help promote regular bowel movements and improve overall digestive health. That said, you're advised to make these changes gradually and consult with a healthcare provider if you experience any severe or persistent symptoms.

The Role of Exercise in Maintaining Healthy Digestion

Overall, regular exercise also plays an important role in promoting healthy digestion and preventing digestive issues such as constipation. If you have any underlying medical conditions, make sure you consult with a healthcare provider before jumping on any exercise program designed to alleviate constipation.

Without further ado, here are ways that exercises can help individuals maintain and alleviate constipation.

1.   Exercise stimulates the muscles in the digestive system

Physical activity stimulates muscles in the digestive system, which, in turn, helps food move through the intestines and prevent constipation. Exercise also helps increase blood flow to the intestines, providing the oxygen and nutrients needed to function properly.

2.   Exercise can help to regulate hormones that affect digestion

Hormones like cortisol and adrenaline affect digestion and have been proven to cause issues such as constipation. Exercise can also help regulate these hormones, reducing stress and improving digestion.

3.   Exercise can help improve gut microbiome

The gut microbiome refers to the collection of bacteria that lives in the digestive system. A healthy gut microbiome is essential for ensuring good digestion and overall health. As expected, regular exercise can improve the diversity and abundance of the gut microbiome, helping maintain healthy digestion.

4.   Increases blood flow

Exercise helps to increase blood flow to the digestive system, which helps to improve the overall health of the digestive system. This increased blood flow can also help to relieve constipation by stimulating the muscles in the colon.

5.   Alleviates stress

The strain of stress can inflict havoc on the digestive system, leading to indigestion, diarrhea, and stomach cramps. Exercise, on the other hand, assuages stress and instills a sense of tranquility, which in turn can enhance the overall health of the digestive system.

6.   Promotes regular bowel movements

Exercise provides a jolt to the muscles within the digestive system, which in turn promotes regular bowel movements. This can stave off constipation and other digestive dilemmas.

Some other exercises that can fuel healthy digestion encompass:

7.   Abdominal exercises

Exercises that target the abdominal muscles, such as crunches and planks, can rev up the digestive system and prompt bowel movements.

8.   Squats

Squats are an exemplary exercise for boosting healthy digestion as they engage the leg and core muscles, which can spark the digestive system.

9.   Cycling

Cycling is a low-impact exercise that can augment healthy digestion by escalating blood flow to the intestines and igniting the digestive system.

10.   Brisk walks

Walking is a low-impact exercise that can promote healthy digestion. Strive to walk energetically for at least 30 minutes daily to invigorate the muscles within the digestive system.

11.   Yoga

Yoga is a mild form of exercise that can mitigate stress and promote healthy digestion. Specific yoga poses, such as the seated forward bend and spinal twist, can be particularly effective in instigating bowel movements.

12.   Aerobic exercise

Aerobic exercises, such as running, swimming, or cycling, can intensify blood flow to the digestive system and boost healthy digestion. Aim to engage in at least 30 minutes of aerobic exercise daily to kindle digestive health.

Techniques for Stress Management to Mitigate Constipation

Stress can take a toll on digestive health, and chronic stress can exacerbate issues such as constipation. Learning to manage stress can reduce the likelihood of constipation and bolster overall digestive health.

Here are some stress management techniques that may be beneficial:

1.   Relaxation maneuvers

Techniques such as deep breathing, meditation, and yoga can mitigate stress and foment relaxation, which can ameliorate digestive health. Deep breathing involves inhaling slowly through the nose and exhaling through the mouth while focusing on the breath and relaxing the body.

Meditation entails focusing the mind on a specific object, thought, or activity while practicing deep breathing and relaxation.

2.   Exercises

Exercise is a natural stress buster and can enhance overall digestive health. As mentioned earlier, exercise propels the muscles in the digestive system, prompting regular bowel movements and reducing the risk of constipation. Regular exercise can also mitigate stress and promote relaxation.

3.   Mind-body therapies

Therapies such as cognitive-behavioral therapy, biofeedback, and hypnotherapy can mitigate stress and improve digestive health. Cognitive-behavioral therapy involves identifying negative thoughts and behaviors that contribute to stress and replacing them with positive ones.

Biofeedback entails using technology to monitor bodily functions such as heart rate and breathing, to regain control over them and mitigate stress. Hypnotherapy involves guided relaxation and visualization techniques to mitigate stress and promote relaxation.

4.   Dietary modifications

Dietary changes, such as abstaining from caffeine and alcohol and increasing fiber intake, can mitigate constipation and enhance digestive health. High-fiber foods such as fruits, vegetables, and whole grains aid in promoting regular bowel movements and preventing constipation.

5. Time management

Poor time management can contribute to stress and elevate the risk of constipation. Learning to manage time effectively and prioritize tasks can mitigate stress and improve digestive health.

If chronic stress or constipation persists, it's imperative to consult a healthcare provider to determine the underlying cause and establish an appropriate treatment plan.

Herbal Remedies and Supplements for Constipation Relief

There are also herbal remedies and supplements that can help to relieve constipation. Here are some to consider:

1.   Psyllium husk

Unleash the power of psyllium, a soluble fiber that can imbue your stool with softness and bulk. Boost your breakfast with oatmeal or smoothies.

2.   Magnesium

Release the tension in your digestive muscles with magnesium, a mineral that can help promote bowel movements. Munch on magnesium-rich spinach or almonds.

3.   Senna

Unleash the digestive tract's mighty muscles with senna, an herbal laxative that can provide relief from constipation. But beware of occasional side effects like cramping and diarrhea.

4.   Probiotics

a.   Nurture your gut health with probiotics, beneficial bacteria that can improve digestion and promote regular bowel movements. Sip on probiotic-rich beverages like kefir or pop a supplement.

5.   Herbal teas

Whisk away constipation with the power of herbal teas like peppermint, ginger, and dandelion. These teas can help stimulate digestion and promote bowel movements.

Remember to use herbal remedies and supplements with care and under the guidance of a healthcare professional.

6.   Aloe vera

Unleash the magic of aloe vera, a natural laxative that can promote regular bowel movements. Use a supplement or try a topical cream or gel.

7.   Castor oil

Kick-start your digestive tract with the gentle power of castor oil, a natural laxative that can stimulate bowel movements. Pop a supplement or use it topically.

8.   Acupressure

Discover the power of acupressure, a technique that involves applying pressure to specific points on the body. Certain acupressure points, like the ones located on the webbing between the thumb and index finger, can help to stimulate the digestive tract and promote regular bowel movements.

Conclusion

In conclusion, natural remedies can be your knight in shining armor when it comes to constipation relief. You can bolster your digestive health by embracing healthy dietary habits, regular exercise, and effective stress management.

Before trying new remedies or supplements, consult your healthcare provider, especially if you have underlying medical conditions or chronic constipation.

Medical Treatment for constipation

Constipation is arguably one of the most common gastrointestinal conditions affecting millions of people around the world. It surfaces when bowel movements inside one's body become difficult or infrequent, thereby causing bloating, discomfort, and other symptoms.

Even though simple lifestyle changes, such as increasing your fiber intakes or exercising can assist in relieving constipation, some people will usually require further medical treatments to treat their slightly severe symptoms. This is what inspired us to create this detailed guide.

Today, we'll discuss various medical treatments for constipation, ranging all the way from over the counter medications to surgeries and medical procedures. We'll also detail some info on the risks, effectiveness, and even potential side effects of each treatment option.

Without further ado, let's jump right in and start by going through some go-to over-the-counter (OTC) medications that could help you manage your constipation.

OTC Medications for Constipation

As with all other sicknesses and conditions, OTC medications are usually the first defense line (in this case treatment) for mild and occasional constipation cases. In such cases, they're usually sufficient in assisting with stool softening as well as stimulating bowel movements in order to make the stool easier pass easier.

With that in mind, let's jump right in and look at some of the most common OTC medications recommended by healthcare experts for constipation relief.

1.   Fiber Supplements

Fiber supplements, such as polycarbophil, methycellulose, and psyllium, will help you boost your stool's bulk in your body, which will, in turn, make it all way easier to pass.

Note that fiber supplements absorb water in your body and swell inside of your intestines, thereby helping move the stool through your digestive tract easier. Also worth noting, generally speaking, these supplements are safe and easy on the body. That said, they have been reported and shown to cause bloating and gas in some individuals.

2.   Osmotic Laxatives

The second in our list is Osmotic laxatives. These laxatives, which include, polyethylene glycol (PEG), magnesium hydroxide and lactulose, also operate in the human body by taking in water in the intestines so they can help soften the stool and stimulate bowel movements.

Like the supplements we've just looked at above, osmotic laxatives' effectiveness is well documented and they're safe for use. That said, they are also known to cause bloating, cramping, and diarrhea in somedividuals.

3.   Stimulant Laxatives

These laxatives, which include bisacodyl and senna, work by first stimulating intestine muscles, thereby in turn helping the stool move faster and easier through your digestive tract. These medicines are normally taken at bedtime so as to induce bowel movements later on at daybreak.

Like most OTC medications, these stimulant laxatives are safe and effective, but in a few cases have been known to result in cramping and diarrhea. When taken in too high doses or for long periods, they could also result in electrolyte imbalances inside the body.

4.   Saline Laxatives

Next, saline laxatives. Like the two medications we've just reviewed, saline laxatives, such as magnesium citrate and magnesium sulfate, heal constipation by taking in water while at the intestines to help soften the stool so bowel movements get initiated. As a general rule of thumb, Saline laxatives are taken orally and they've been so effective, such that some of them are reported to help initiate bowel movements in a few hours.

5.   Stool Softeners

Softeners, like docusate sodium, heal mild constipations by drawing the water in your body to the stool, making it easier to go through. That said, while these medicines are usually safe and well-tolerated, they don't always work as fast as most other constipation medications and may sometimes take up to several days to produce bowel movements.

There you have it, the detailed list of a few of the best OTC medications for relieving constipation. Remember, it's essential to follow all the instructions of the medications as detailed on their packages. And you should not take them longer than recommended.

Remember, prolonged usage of these medications (even though they're OTC) can not only result in dependence, but it has also proven to worsen constipation over time. Also remember to consult with a trusted healthcare professional before committing to any medication, especially if you currently have other conditions or are taking other types of medications.

The Best Prescription Medications for Prolonged Constipations

For individuals suffering from enduring constipation, OTC treatments may not be enough to offer any relief. In such cases, an even better option would be to go for prescription treatments to manage the chronic symptoms.

Let's look at a few common kinds of prescription medicines for chronic constipations recommended by most healthcare experts today.

1.   Lubiprostone

This medicine helps boost the amount of fluids in your intestines, which in turn, helps soften your stool and induces bowel movements. Lubiprostone is currently approved to treat chronic idiopathic constipation as well as irritable bowel syndrome with constipation in adults.

That said, while lubiprostone is well tolerated and safe, it can result in abdominal pain, diarrhea, and nausea in some individuals.

2.   Linaclotide

This is a constipation medication that works through increasing the amounts of secretion of fluids in your intestines, while simultaneously reducing pain signals from the intestine's nerves. Like Lubiprostone, it is approved to treat irritable bowel syndrome with constipation and chronic idiopathic constipation in patients of varying ages.

Reported side effects linked to using the medication to relieve constipation are bloating, abdominal pain, and diarrhea.

3.   Plecanatide

Plecanatide follows the same trend you must've noticed with a wide array constipation medications so-far, i.e. it relieves constipation by increasing fluids secretion in your intestines, thereby helping soften your stool and induce bowel movements.

The medication is approved for chronic idiopathic constipation treatment in adults. It's also well-tolerated and safe to consume. That said, it can result in some mild abdominal pain and diarrhea in some.

4.   Tegaserod

Manufactured for the relief of constipation as well as IRS (irritable bowel syndrome), Tegaserod is a 5-HT that'll work by stimulating muscles in your intestines and reducing pain signals from the intestines' nerves.

It's approved for treating irritable bowel syndrome with constipation in women and chronic idiopathic constipation.

Unfortunately, this constipation medicine has been linked to increased risks of heart attack and stroke. That is why it's only available through a restricted distribution program.

Generally speaking, prescription medications designed to relieve chronic constipation must only be consumed under the supervision of a healthcare expert. The reason is simple – some of them might not be appropriate for everyone and could cause some side effects or adversely interact with any other medications one might be taking. Remember to consult with a healthcare expert before starting new medications.

Medical Procedures

In more severe cases, medical procedures may be needed to treat and diagnose constipation caused by underlying medical conditions or anatomical abnormalities. Below, we'll look at a few common medical procedures that can be utilized to manage constipation:

1.   Colonoscopy

Colonoscopies are medical procedures involving the use of long, flexible tubes with cameras at one end in order to examine the insides of the colon. Around the world, doctors use it to identify any abnormalities or blockages that could be behind the constipation. During the procedure, healthcare providers may also retrieve tissue samples or remove polyps. These usually aid in further testing.

Generally speaking, colonoscopies are safe, with the worst complaints being the fact it can result in some discomfort and rare complications like bleeding or perforation of the large intestines.

2.   Anorectal manometry

This is a test doctors use to measure the muscle strength and pressure in the anal sphincter and rectum. Doctors worldwide use anorectal manometry to diagnose problems linked to bowel movements, and that includes serious constipation cases.

Amidst the anorectal medical procedure, a small and flexible tube is inserted into one's rectum. To quantity the pressure, the Doctor will then ask the individual to squeeze or relax their muscles.

This medical procedure is also generally safe and well-tolerated. The only downside is it can cause some discomfort.

3.   Biofeedback

Biofeedbacks are a kind of therapy where doctors utilize sensors to watch and measure muscle activity around the pelvic floor then provide feedback to their patients. In constipation patients, it's also utilized to help the patients know how to control their bowel movements as well as improve their ability to easily pass stool.

That said, while Biofeedback is generally well-tolerated and safe like most other medical procedures we've seen, it can take several sessions to before one sees the results.

4.   Fecal transplant

Fecal transplant, also called fecal microbiota transplantation (FMT), is a procedure that involves transferring fecal matter from healthy donors into the constipation patient's gastrointestinal tract. For decades, this procedure was used to restore the balance of healthy bacteria in the gut while also treating conditions like Clostridium difficile infection.

Just remember that fecal transplant can cause some discomfort and there will be a small risk of infection.

5.   Surgery

Surgery will only be needed in rare constipation cases that have been caused by anatomical abnormalities like bowel obstruction, anal fissures, or rectal prolapse. Surgeries in these situations may involve removing or repairing damaged tissue and rerouting one's digestive system in order to bypass the affected region.

Complications and risks associated with these kinds of surgeries are obvious, and they include bleeding, infection, or bowel perforation.

While all the treatments we've reviewed above will effectively relieve constipation, they all also have their potential risks as well as side effects worth noting.

Common side effects of using laxatives and prescription medications for constipation include:

- Electrolyte imbalances

- Dehydration

- Nausea

- Diarrhea

- Abdominal cramping

In extremely rare cases, both medications could also result in more serious complications, like:

- Profuse bleeding

- Perforation of the bowel

- Infection

Let's dive deeper into risks and potential side effects associated with every medical treatment we've mentioned above.

Remember, the likelihood and severity of the side effects varies significantly, dependent upon your individual health status, the treatment you've used, and other factors.

That's why it's essential to discuss the potential benefits and risks of any medical treatment you're considering with a healthcare expert you trust before beginning any of the actual treatments. Constipation patients ought to also beware of any pre- or post-procedure instructions. This will minimize their complication risks.

Remember, in most situations, benefits of the treatment will outweigh the risks. That said, as a patient, you still should be fully informed before making any decisions about your healthcare.

Conclusion

Constipation is, without a doubt, a frustrating and uncomfortable condition, but, luckily, there are various medical treatments available to help alleviate symptoms. Over-the-counter (OTC) laxatives should be efficient for short-term relief, while prescription medications and medical procedures might be needed for serious and chronic constipations.

That said, while these treatments are often effective, it's still important that you discuss the benefits and risks with a healthcare expert and be aware of potential risks and side effects. With the ideal treatment plan, it's possible to manage even chronic constipation and improve bowel function without a hassle.

Lifestyle Changes to Prevent Constipation

Constipation afflicts many individuals at some point in their lives, causing a backlog of fecal matter, difficulty with defecation, and infrequent bowel movements. Factors like insufficient fiber consumption, dehydration, sedentary behavior, and certain medications can all trigger constipation.

Luckily, a slew of lifestyle alterations can improve digestion and prevent this predicament al-together.

This guide will explore 15 lifestyle changes that can keep constipation at bay. These changes include upping your fiber intake, hydrating amply, exercising regularly, and shunning constipation-provoking foods.

We will also delve into the positive effects of probiotic-rich foods like kefir and yogurt on digestion. By adhering to these easy lifestyle adjustments, you can ameliorate your digestion and stave off the unpleasantness and inconvenience of constipation.

1.   Boost Your Fiber Intake

Fiber is an indispensable nutrient for digestive health, adding bulk to stool and facilitating its painless passage through the digestive system. Soluble fiber dissolves in water, forming a gel-like substance that retards digestion. Insoluble fiber doesn't dissolve in water and augments stool bulk. For optimum digestive health, it's vital to consume both types of fiber.

Oats, beans, peas, lentils, fruits, and vegetables are excellent sources of soluble fiber, while whole grains, nuts, seeds, and veggies such as broccoli, carrots, and celery contain insoluble fiber.

2.   Hydrate Ample

Adequate hydration is vital for digestive health and bowel function. Water mollifies stool, making it easier to pass. It also averts dehydration, which can exacerbate constipation. Aim to drink at least eight glasses of water per day. If plain water doesn't appeal to you, add cucumber or lemon slices to flavor it.

3.   Exercise Regularly

Exercise is fundamental to overall health and can also thwart constipation. It stimulates the intestinal muscles, facilitating the movement of stool through the digestive tract. Regular exercise can also alleviate stress, which can contribute to constipation. Try to work out for at least 30 minutes every day, engaging in moderate activities like brisk walking, cycling, or swimming.

4.   Don't Hold in Stool

Retaining stool can trigger constipation, as the stool becomes harder and drier, making it trickier to evacuate. If you feel the urge to go, don't delay. Head to the bathroom immediately. Try to relax, allowing the stool to pass naturally without straining.

5.   Establish Regular Bathroom Habits

Creating a routine for bathroom breaks can prevent constipation. Try to defecate at the same time every day, preferably following a meal. This trains your body to expect a bowel movement at a specific time and can assist in relaxation rather than rushing or forcing a bowel movement.

6.   Avoid Laxatives

Laxatives can temporarily alleviate constipation, but they should only be used under the supervision of a healthcare professional. Overusing laxatives can lead to dependence and exacerbate constipation. Certain types of laxatives can also cause dehydration or imbalances in electrolytes. If you're considering using a laxative, consult your healthcare provider first.

7.   Limit Processed Foods

Processed foods are often low in fiber and high in fat, sugar, and salt, which can slow down the digestive process and lead to constipation. To avoid constipation, strive to restrict processed foods and opt for whole, unprocessed foods instead. Examples of processed foods include fast food, chips, candy, and frozen meals.

8.   Indulge in Probiotic-Rich Delicacies

Probiotics, the living microorganisms, can bestow a plethora of health benefits when consumed judiciously. These friendly bacteria can aid in promoting digestive health and thwarting constipation. They work their magic by harmonizing the gut's bacteria, which results in regulating bowel movements and obviating digestive discomfort.

Some probiotic-rich delicacies that can be added to your diet include yogurt, kefir, sauerkraut, kimchi, and kombucha. These lip-smacking foods harbor live cultures of beneficial bacteria that can help in promoting healthy digestion. Yogurt and kefir, in particular, are excellent sources of probiotics as they contain strains of bacteria that are specifically beneficial for digestive health.

In addition to probiotic-rich foods, prebiotic foods can also be advantageous in preventing constipation. Prebiotics, a type of fiber, serve as food for the beneficial bacteria present in the gut. Some prebiotic-rich foods that can be added to your diet include garlic, onions, bananas, asparagus, and oats.

It is crucial to note that not all probiotic supplements and products are equivalent in effectiveness. It is recommended to choose products that have undergone quality testing and proven to be effective. When considering a probiotic supplement, you must consult a healthcare professional to determine the best option for your needs.

9. Sufficient Sleep is Vital

Adequate sleep is essential for overall health, including digestive health. Inadequate sleep can contribute to stress, leading to constipation. Aim for at least seven hours of sleep per night. To improve sleep quality, establish a regular sleep schedule, avoid caffeine and alcohol before bed, and create a soothing bedtime routine.

10. Steer Clear of Dairy Products

Dairy products can trigger constipation in some people, especially those who are lactose intolerant or sensitive to dairy. Lactose, a sugar found in milk and dairy products, can cause digestive discomfort and symptoms like bloating, gas, and constipation when the body cannot break it down.

In addition to lactose, dairy products can also be high in fat and low in fiber. These factors can contribute to constipation by slowing the digestive process and making it arduous for stool to pass through the colon. Cheese and cream, high-fat dairy products, are particularly problematic for constipation.

11. Manage Stress Effectively

Stress can wreak havoc on digestive health. It can cause the muscles in the digestive system to contract, leading to constipation. To prevent constipation, it is imperative to manage stress effectively. This can include practicing relaxation techniques such as deep breathing, meditation, or yoga. Regular exercise, sufficient sleep, and establishing a routine can also help reduce stress levels.

12.   Avoid Certain Medications

Some medications can contribute to constipation. These include pain medications, such as opioids, antacids containing aluminum and calcium, and certain antidepressants. If you are taking a drug causing constipation, talk to your healthcare provider about alternatives or ways to manage the side effects.

13.   Boost Magnesium Intake

Magnesium, a mineral that plays a crucial role in muscle and nerve function, including the muscles in the intestine, can help prevent constipation. Foods high in magnesium include leafy green vegetables, nuts, seeds, and whole grains.

Magnesium supplements are also available, but it is best to talk to your healthcare provider before taking them.

14.   Stay Hydrated

Dehydration can exacerbate constipation by making the stool harder and more challenging to pass. To prevent dehydration, drink plenty of water and avoid beverages that can contribute to dehydration, such as caffeine and alcohol. Eating foods high in water content, such as fruits and vegetables, can also help prevent dehydration.

15.   Seek Medical Assistance for Chronic Constipation

If you are experiencing chronic constipation, it is imperative to seek medical attention. Chronic constipation is defined as having fewer than three bowel movements per week for at least three months.

Your healthcare provider can help determine the underlying cause of your constipation and suggest appropriate treatment options. Treatment options may include dietary changes, medication, or other therapies.

16.   Maintain a Balanced Weight

Maintaining a healthy weight is essential for overall health, including digestive health. Being overweight or obese can contribute to constipation by putting pressure on the intestines and slowing the digestive process. Aim for a balanced diet and regular exercise to maintain a healthy weight.

Age-Specific Lifestyle Changes That Can Help With Constipation

Yes, there are specific life changes that men, women, and children can make to deal with constipation. Here are some suggestions:

For Men and Women

- **Boost Your Fiber Intake**

By consuming a wide variety of high-fiber foods, you can significantly enhance your digestive health, promote regular bowel movements, and ensure that your gastrointestinal system stays in optimal condition. Aim for 25 grams of fiber daily through fruits, veggies, whole grains, and legumes.

- **Stay Adequately Hydrated**

Ensuring that you consume a sufficient amount of water on a regular basis is crucial in maintaining proper hydration levels, which in turn aids in the softening of your stool and facilitates its effortless passage. Drink eight cups of water every day.

- **Engage in Regualr Exercise**

By engaging in regular exercise, which involves consistent physical activity, you can significantly enhance and stimulate your digestive system's functionality by increasing the blood flow to your intestines, ultimately leading to better overall health and well-being. It is highly recommended that you strive to engage in physical activity for a minimum of 30 minutes on a daily basis for the majority of the week.

- **Respond to Your Urge to Poo**

Ignoring the urge to defecate causes constipation. It is of utmost importance that you pay close attention to the signals your body is sending you and act accordingly by promptly going to attend to its needs.

- **Avoid Breath-holding**

Don't hold your breath while straining to pass stool as it can worsen constipation. While you are seated on the toilet, it is recommended that you take slow, deep, and natural breaths in order to promote relaxation and ease any discomfort.

For Children

- **Promote Healthy Eating**

Children should eat fruits, veggies, whole grains, and lean proteins for a healthy diet.

- **Establish a Regular Bathroom Routine**

Encourage your child to establish a regular bathroom routine, like going after meals.

- **Encourage Physical Activity**

In order to further promote regular bowel movements, it is highly recommended that you motivate your child to engage in physical activity on a daily basis.

- **Limit Processed Foods**

It is highly recommended to limit the consumption of processed foods as they are often lacking in fiber, which can lead to constipation and other digestive issues. It is highly recommended that you motivate and inspire your offspring to consume nutrient-dense, unrefined meals.

- **Offer Plenty of Fluids**

Offer as much fluids as possilble to your kids so it can keep stool soft and make it easy to pass.

In addition to these lifestyle changes, it is vital to consult a healthcare provider if constipation persists or is severe.

Conclusion

Conclusively, constipation can be a vexing and discomforting predicament. However, you can take several lifestyle measures to prevent it. Boosting your fiber intake, staying hydrated, exercising regularly, establishing regular bathroom habits, and avoiding stool retention are practical ways to prevent this predicament.

Furthermore, managing stress, avoiding certain medications, increasing magnesium intake, and seeking medical attention if you experience chronic constipation are essential steps in preventing and treating constipation. These lifestyle changes will help maintain healthy bowel functions and ensure constipation does not interfere with your daily life.

Coping with chronic constipation

Chronic constipation plagues countless individuals across the globe, causing a substantial strain in these individual's daily lives. This affliction is characterized by infrequent defecation, accompanied by arduous stool passing and straining. Regarding the root causes of chronic constipation, they are multifarious, ranging from dietary habits and medication intake to stress and underlying medical conditions.

Even worse, the management of chronic constipation can be a daunting task, with both physical and emotional challenges to overcome. Keep reading this blog post to unearth innovative tactics for coping with the emotional toll of chronic constipation, combating the social stigma associated with this condition, and discovering support and resources to combat this affliction.

Strategies for Managing the Emotional Impact of Chronic Constipation

Chronic constipation can harm one's emotional balance. It can cause debilitating symptoms through pressure, agitation, and fluster, creating a vicious cycle. Effective strategies are crucial for managing the emotional impact of chronic constipation. Listed below are a few atypical methods for effectively managing the emotional repercussions that arise from experiencing chronic constipation.

1.   Validate and articulate your emotions

It is of utmost importance that you take the time to acknowledge, understand, and effectively communicate your emotions in a manner that is authentic and true to yourself. In order to effectively manage the emotional impact of chronic constipation, it is imperative to first acknowledge, validate, and clearly articulate the complex range of emotions that one may experience.

Remember, constipation is frustrating, embarrassing, and isolating. Realizing and accepting these sentiments is imperative. By taking the time to consciously identify and validate your feelings, you can cultivate a greater understanding of yourself and ultimately establish successful strategies for managing and navigating through challenging situations.

2.   Practice stress-alleviating techniques

Engage in various stress-alleviating techniques on a regular basis to enhance your overall well-being and reduce the negative impact of stress on your physical and mental health. Stress worsens constipation and damages emotions.

By consistently engaging in stress-alleviating practices such as transcendental meditation, mindfulness, or Tai Chi, individuals can effectively decrease their stress levels and experience a heightened sense of relaxation.

3.   Stay physically engaged

It is highly recommended that you remain actively involved in physical activities to maintain your overall health and well-being. Exercise can aid in bowel movements and regularity. It reduces stress and improves emotional well-being. Rock climbing, skateboarding, or parkour can help manage the emotional impact of chronic constipation.

4.   Incorporate unconventional relaxation techniques

Incorporate a wide range of unique and innovative relaxation techniques that deviate from the norm and challenge traditional methods. By exploring alternative methods of relaxation such as lucid dreaming, sensory deprivation, or sound healing, individuals can effectively alleviate stress and promote relaxation in ways that deviate from traditional practices. Practice these techniques at home or with a healthcare provider's guidance.

5.   Use affirmative self-talk

Employ positive and encouraging language when speaking to oneself. The act of engaging in negative self-talk, which involves speaking to oneself in a critical and pessimistic manner, has the potential to worsen the symptoms of constipation and cause damage to one's emotional state of being. Positive self-talk reduces stress and promotes a better outlook by reciting mantras or focusing on goals.

6.   Seek professional counsel

It is highly recommended that you seek the advice and guidance of a qualified and experienced professional in the relevant field to assist you in making informed decisions and achieving your desired outcomes.

Some may need professional help to manage chronic constipation's emotional impact. Providers can help manage stress and anxiety related to constipation and suggest therapy or interventions for emotional well-being.

Dealing With the Social Stigma of Constipation

The social stigma of constipation can confound even the most resolute individuals, as it is often perceived as a shameful and taboo topic. Those who suffer from chronic constipation may feel isolated and despondent, resulting in a diminished quality of life and negative emotions. Nonetheless, there are effective methods to surmount the social stigma of constipation and obtain support and understanding from others.

To overcome the social stigma of constipation, it is essential to enlighten yourself and others about the condition. Misconceptions and negative attitudes may arise since many people are unaware of the causes and symptoms of constipation. By educating yourself and spreading that awareness to others, you can help diminish the stigma and foster comprehension.

Furthermore, it is crucial to shun feelings of humiliation or embarrassment because of having constipation. Recognize that constipation is a widespread condition that affects millions of individuals across the world, regardless of age, gender, or socioeconomic status.

Instead of feeling ashamed, it can be advantageous to acknowledge your condition candidly and sincerely, whether with loved ones, a support group, or a healthcare provider. In doing so, you may discover that others are more compassionate and accepting than you initially thought.

Seeking support from others can also be a valuable way to cope with the social stigma of constipation. Engaging in conversations with friends, family, or a support group about your condition can provide a sense of validation and understanding. Connecting with others who have undergone similar challenges and exchanging coping strategies and tips can also be beneficial.

Lastly, seeking healthcare providers or resources knowledgeable about constipation can be helpful and provide guidance and support. Numerous organizations, such as the International Foundation for Gastrointestinal Disorders (IFFGD), offer educational resources and support networks for individuals with constipation.

Additionally, collaborating with a healthcare provider conversant with constipation and its treatment alternatives can help you manage your symptoms and feel more confident in your ability to cope with the condition.

Finding Support and Resources for Managing Constipation

Discovering support and resources to manage constipation is crucial in handling this condition. These avenues can offer direction, enlightenment, and a sense of validation and empathy, which can aid in managing the emotional and social impact of chronic constipation.

Here are some novel suggestions for finding support and resources to manage constipation:

1.   Consult a healthcare provider

One of the most impactful ways to seek support and resources for managing constipation is to consult a healthcare provider. Healthcare professionals can enlighten you on the root cause of constipation, identify any underlying medical issues, and propose treatment options.

They can also provide informative resources and link you with other healthcare specialists such as dietitians or physical therapists, who can assist in managing your symptoms.

2.   Connect with patient support organizations

Patient support organizations such as the International Foundation for Gastrointestinal Disorders (IFFGD) avail resources and support for individuals grappling with constipation.

These organizations can provide educational materials, support groups, and online forums where you can connect with others who have experienced similar challenges. Moreover, some organizations offer helplines manned by knowledgeable volunteers who can answer questions and offer guidance.

3.   Explore online resources

Numerous online resources are available to provide educational materials, support, and guidance for managing constipation. Websites like WebMD, Mayo Clinic, and Healthline offer comprehensive information on constipation, its causes, and treatment options.

Social media platforms such as Facebook and Twitter can also be a source of support and community for individuals grappling with constipation.

4.   Talk to loved ones

Talking to loved ones such as family members or close friends can provide a sense of validation and empathy when coping with constipation. Loved ones can offer emotional support, help with daily activities, and encouragement when dealing with the challenges of constipation.

5.   Consider therapy

For some individuals, therapy can help manage the emotional impact of chronic constipation. Cognitive-behavioral therapy (CBT) can help individuals identify negative thought patterns and develop coping strategies for managing stress and anxiety related to constipation.

Additionally, psychotherapy can provide a safe space to discuss the challenges of constipation and develop strategies for managing the condition.

- National Institute of Diabetes and Digestive and Kidney Diseases (NIDDK)

The NIDDK is a part of the National Institutes of Health (NIH) that provides resources and information on digestive diseases and conditions, including constipation.

Their website offers a wealth of information on the causes, symptoms, and treatment options for constipation, as well as resources for managing the emotional impact of the condition.

- International Foundation for Gastrointestinal Disorders (IFFGD)

The IFFGD is a non-profit organization that provides support, education, and advocacy for people with gastrointestinal disorders, including chronic constipation.

Their website offers information on treatment options, lifestyle changes, coping strategies for managing constipation, and resources for finding support and connecting with others going through similar experiences.

- American Gastroenterological Association (AGA)

The AGA is a professional organization of gastroenterologists that provides information and resources on digestive diseases and conditions, including constipation.

Their website offers information on the causes, symptoms, and treatment options for constipation and resources for finding a gastroenterologist in your area.

- Patient Advocacy Organizations

Many patient advocacy organizations focus on specific conditions, including chronic constipation. These organizations can provide resources, support, and advocacy for people with constipation, as well as opportunities to connect with others who are going through similar experiences.

Age-specific methods for coping with chronic constipation:

As promised at the beginning of the guide, let's jump right and look at some age-specific methods for coping with chronic constipation.

We've categorized these into three distinct sections, men, women, and children.

Men

To diminish the peril of chronic constipation, men must integrate a high-fiber diet, regular exercise, and ample hydration into their routine.

To avoid straining during bowel movements, men must refrain from exerting unnecessary pressure, and if the symptoms persist, they must seek medical aid to handle the issue.

Women

Due to the hormonal changes that take place during the menstrual cycle or pregnancy, women are more vulnerable to constipation. Women must maintain a healthy diet, exercise regularly, and consume generous amounts of fluids to prevent this condition.

They must also confer with their healthcare provider regarding medications' potential contribution to constipation and explore non-pharmacological alternatives.

Children

Chronic constipation in children is a daunting obstacle to surmount. Parents can assist their children in coping with this condition by urging them to consume a healthy, fiber-rich diet, stay hydrated, and exercise regularly.

Furthermore, establishing a consistent toileting routine and abstaining from withholding could enhance bowel function. Parents must also consult their child's healthcare provider to explore treatment options if their child has chronic constipation.

Conclusion

In conclusion, chronic constipation is a physically and emotionally taxing condition. However, by maintaining a positive outlook, implementing relaxation techniques, exercising regularly, documenting food intake, and seeking support from family, friends, or support groups, individuals can better cope with the emotional strain of this condition.

Additionally, by utilizing resources such as the NIDDK, IFFGD, or AGA, individuals can access valuable support to manage the situation effectively. Remember, you are not alone, and help is available to assist you as you manage your chronic constipation.

The Connection Between Constipation and Other Health Conditions

Constipation is a ubiquitous gastrointestinal condition that impacts people of all ages - from wee babes to the elderly. It is marked by infrequent excretions or trouble expelling fecal matter and may be accompanied by abdominal agony, inflation, and discomfort. Although sporadic constipation is normal and usually not a cause for alarm, persistent or severe obstruction can drastically impact the quality of life. It may be an indication of an underlying medical ailment.

As a matter of fact, constipation is frequently intertwined with other medical conditions and may even be an indication of an underlying disorder. Deciphering the link between obstruction and these medical conditions can help individuals better manage their symptoms and seek appropriate treatment when necessary.

In this article, we will scrutinize some of the most common health conditions connected to obstruction, as well as other conditions that may cause or exacerbate obstruction. By augmenting our awareness of the potential links between obstruction and other health problems, we can take proactive measures to promote our overall health and well-being.

Health conditions connected to constipation

Let's plunge into the depths of this condition and uncover some of the most prevalent health conditions linked to constipation, illuminating their underlying mechanisms and potential courses of action.

1.   Irritable bowel syndrome (IBS)

IBS is a chronic digestive disorder that can trigger various symptoms, including constipation, diarrhea, abdominal pain, and bloating. In some cases of IBS, the muscles in the colon can sluggishly or vigorously contract, producing constipation.

Conversely, the muscles can contract too briskly, leading to diarrhea. Treatment for constipation linked to IBS may involve tinkering with one's diet, such as increasing fiber intake or avoiding certain trigger foods. Additionally, medications that regulate bowel function, like laxatives or antispasmodics, may prove useful.

2.   Hypothyroidism

Hypothyroidism occurs when the thyroid gland fails to generate adequate thyroid hormone, which can decelerate many bodily functions, including digestion. Constipation is a typical sign of hypothyroidism, in addition to fatigue, weight gain, and dry skin.

Treating constipation associated with hypothyroidism may require hormone replacement therapy to normalize thyroid hormone levels. Dietary modifications and medications to regulate bowel function may also help.

3.   Sedentary lifestyle

A lack of physical activity and a sedentary lifestyle can also contribute to constipation. Exercise animates the muscles in the digestive tract and promotes regular bowel movements. Conversely, sitting for long periods, like during an extended flight or workday, can impede bowel movements and contribute to constipation.

Treatment for constipation linked to a sedentary lifestyle may involve increasing physical activity, taking breaks to move around during lengthy periods of sitting, and making dietary adjustments.

4.   Colon cancer

Colon cancer can cause constipation as a symptom, albeit less often than other causes. In colon cancer, a tumor can entirely or partially obstruct the colon, causing constipation, abdominal pain, and bloating. Other symptoms of colon cancer may include rectal bleeding, weight loss, and fatigue.

Treatment for constipation associated with colon cancer may vary depending on the tumor's stage. It may include surgery, chemotherapy, radiation therapy, and medications to relieve constipation symptoms.

5.   Eating disorders

Eating disorders, such as anorexia nervosa or bulimia, can induce constipation due to insufficient food intake and dehydration. Also, using laxatives as a purging method can contribute to constipation.

Treatment for constipation linked to eating disorders may involve nutritional counseling, hydration therapy, bowel retraining, and addressing the underlying eating disorder.

6.   Inflammatory bowel disease (IBD)

IBD is a persistent inflammatory disorder of the digestive tract, comprising Crohn's disease and ulcerative colitis. Constipation may occur in some cases of IBD, although diarrhea is a more common symptom. In IBD, inflammation can disrupt the normal function of the digestive tract, resulting in changes in bowel habits and difficulty passing stool.

Treatment for constipation linked to IBD may involve medications that regulate bowel function, like laxatives or prokinetic agents. Additionally, dietary adjustments such as avoiding trigger foods or following a low-residue diet during flare-ups may be helpful. In severe cases, surgery may be necessary to remove damaged portions of the digestive tract.

7.   Parkinson's disease

The nerves and muscles that control bowel function are mercilessly ravaged by Parkinson's disease, resulting in constipation. This symptom may manifest years before tremors or stiffness set in. Parkinson's disease renders the digestive tract muscles rigid and sluggish, causing constipation.

To combat this, treatment options may involve drugs that activate bowel movement like prokinetic agents or laxatives. Prescriptions of dietary changes and exercise may also be recommended to promote regular bowel function.

8.   Multiple sclerosis (MS)

MS is a chronic autoimmune disease that attacks the central nervous system, including the nerves that regulate bowel function. Constipation is a common symptom of MS and can be triggered by various factors such as muscle weakness or spasticity, and side effects of medication.

To mitigate constipation associated with MS, dietary modifications such as increasing fiber intake, avoiding certain trigger foods, and medications that promote bowel movement like prokinetic agents or laxatives may be recommended.

9.   Diabetes

Diabetes is a chronic metabolic disorder that impedes the body's ability to produce or respond to insulin. Constipation is a common symptom of diabetes, especially when blood sugar levels are poorly regulated. High blood sugar levels can damage the nerves responsible for bowel function, leading to constipation.

To address this, dietary changes like increasing fiber intake or avoiding trigger foods may be prescribed. Healthcare providers may also administer medications that promote bowel movement like prokinetic agents or laxatives.

10.   Pregnancy

Hormonal changes and the pressure of a growing uterus on the digestive tract can trigger constipation during pregnancy. This symptom is particularly prevalent during the later stages of pregnancy. To alleviate constipation associated with pregnancy, dietary modifications like increasing fiber intake and staying hydrated may be recommended.

Gentle exercise, too, may be prescribed to promote regular bowel function. In some cases, healthcare providers may recommend the use of laxatives or stool softeners.

Other health conditions that may cause or worsen constipation

In addition to the health conditions directly linked to constipation, a plethora of other factors may instigate or exacerbate this unpleasant ailment. Some of these factors interfere with the nerves, muscles, or other systems implicated in bowel function.

Conversely, others instigate dehydration or electrolyte imbalances that impact the consistency of stool and hinder bowel movement. In this section, we shall delve into some of the most common health conditions that can trigger or intensify constipation, elucidating the underlying mechanisms and potential remedies.

1.   Dehydration

Dehydration can parch your stool, rendering it rigid and arduous to evacuate. It is critical to guzzle enough water to sustain soft and facile stool passage. Furthermore, caffeine and alcohol consumption can fuel dehydration and exacerbate constipation.

2.   Medications

A plethora of medications can ignite constipation as a side effect, including painkillers, antidepressants, and antacids. If you are suffering from constipation as a side effect of drugs, discuss alternative treatments or medication adjustments with your healthcare provider.

3.   Sedentary lifestyle

A dearth of physical activity and a sedentary lifestyle can also contribute to constipation. Exercise invigorates the muscles in the digestive tract and promotes regular bowel movements.

Additionally, prolonged periods of sitting, such as during a lengthy flight or workday, can retard bowel movements and exacerbate constipation.

4.   Colon cancer

Constipation often manifests as a symptom of colon cancer, although it is less frequent than other causes. In colon cancer, a tumor can partially or fully obstruct the colon, leading to constipation, abdominal pain, and bloating.

Other symptoms of colon cancer may include rectal bleeding, weight loss, and fatigue. Consult with your healthcare provider if you experience persistent alterations in bowel habits or other symptoms of colon cancer.

5.   Eating disorders

Eating disorders, such as anorexia nervosa or bulimia, can instigate constipation due to inadequate food intake and dehydration. Moreover, employing laxatives as a means of purging can exacerbate constipation.

Treatment for constipation associated with eating disorders may encompass nutritional counseling, hydration therapy, and bowel retraining.

6.   Inflammatory bowel disease (IBD)

IBD is a chronic inflammatory disorder of the digestive tract, encompassing Crohn's disease and ulcerative colitis. Constipation can arise in some cases of IBD, albeit diarrhea is a more common symptom.

In IBD, inflammation can disrupt the conventional function of the digestive tract, leading to alterations in bowel habits and difficulty passing stool. Treatment for constipation associated with IBD may include medications that regulate bowel function, such as laxatives or prokinetic agents, as well as dietary modifications.

Conclusion

Ultimately, constipation plagues the gastrointestinal tract and can be instigated or intensified by an array of health maladies, prescriptions, and habits of life. Uncovering the root causes of constipation and collaborating with a medical professional to create an individualized course of action can alleviate symptoms and elevate one's standard of living.

If you find yourself subject to persistent constipation or alterations to your bowel routine, seeking an assessment and fitting therapy from a healthcare provider is absolutely crucial.